H. PYLORI TREATMENT HANDBOOK FOR BEGINNERS

The Basic Guide to Diagnosing, Causes, Symptoms, Foods to Avoid, Prevention, Treatment, and When to See a Doctor

Dr. Nina Jespersen

Table of Contents

INTRODUCTION TO H. PYLORI

Overview Of H. Pylori

Definition And Description Of Helicobacter Pylori (H. Pylori)

Significance Of H. Pylori In Gastrointestinal Health

Goals Of The Book

Purpose Of The Book

To Provide A Thorough Guide On Diagnosing And Treating H. Pylori Infections

To Offer Practical Advice For Patients And Healthcare Providers

How To Use This Book

Overview Of The Book's Structure

Tips For Navigating The Content

Helicobacter pylori (H. pylori) is a gram-negative bacterium that plays a significant role in various gastrointestinal disorders. Understanding this pathogen is crucial for effective diagnosis, treatment, and management of related conditions. This introduction will outline what H. pylori is, its impact on gastrointestinal health, the goals of this book, and how to best use the information provided.

1. Overview Of H. Pylori

A. Definition And Description Of Helicobacter Pylori

What is H. pylori?

Definition: Helicobacter pylori is a type of bacteria that infects the stomach lining. It is spiral-shaped and possesses flagella that allow it to move through the viscous environment of the stomach.

Characteristics: H. pylori is unique in its ability to survive in the acidic environment of the stomach, where it creates a less acidic microenvironment around itself. This is facilitated by its production of urease, an enzyme that breaks down urea into ammonia, which neutralizes stomach acid.

Infection Mechanism:

Transmission: The exact mode of transmission is not fully understood, but it is believed to spread through contaminated food, water, or direct contact with saliva or fecal matter.

Colonization: Once H. pylori reaches the stomach lining, it adheres to the gastric epithelium and causes chronic inflammation, which can lead to more serious conditions if left untreated.

B. Significance Of H. Pylori In Gastrointestinal Health

Associated Conditions:

Peptic Ulcers: H. pylori is a major cause of peptic ulcers, which are sores that develop on the lining of the stomach, small intestine, or esophagus.

Chronic Gastritis: Chronic infection can lead to chronic gastritis, characterized by inflammation of the stomach lining.

Gastric Cancer: Long-term infection with H. pylori is a risk factor for gastric cancer, particularly in individuals with a family history or other predisposing factors.

Prevalence:

Global Reach: H. pylori infection is widespread, affecting a significant portion of the global population. It is particularly common in developing countries due to poorer sanitation and hygiene.

Impact on Quality of Life:

Symptoms: Infection can lead to symptoms such as abdominal pain, bloating, nausea, and frequent burping, which can affect daily activities and quality of life.

C. Goals Of The Book

Comprehensive Guide:

Diagnosis and Treatment: The primary goal of this book is to provide a thorough guide on diagnosing and treating H. pylori infections. This includes understanding diagnostic tests, treatment regimens, and management strategies.

Up-to-Date Information: The book aims to present the most current research, guidelines, and practices in the field of H. pylori management.

Practical Advice:

For Patients: Offer practical advice for patients on how to manage their condition, including dietary recommendations, lifestyle changes, and understanding treatment options.

For Healthcare Providers: Provide healthcare professionals with detailed information on diagnosis, treatment protocols, and patient management strategies to ensure effective care.

2. Purpose Of The Book

A. To Provide A Thorough Guide On Diagnosing And Treating H. Pylori Infections

Diagnostic Approaches:

Tests and Procedures: Detailed explanations of various diagnostic tests used to identify H. pylori, such as breath tests, stool tests, blood tests, and endoscopic biopsy.

Treatment Options:

Antibiotic Therapy: Information on current antibiotic regimens used to eradicate H. pylori, including the choice of antibiotics and potential combinations.

Acid Suppression Therapy: Description of medications used to reduce stomach acid and enhance the effectiveness of antibiotic treatment.

B. To Offer Practical Advice For Patients And Healthcare Providers

Patient Management:

Symptom Relief: Strategies for managing symptoms and minimizing discomfort during and after treatment.

Diet and Lifestyle: Recommendations for dietary adjustments and lifestyle changes that can help in managing the condition and supporting treatment.

Healthcare Provider Guidance:

Treatment Protocols: Guidance on creating effective treatment plans and monitoring patient progress.

Patient Education: Tips on educating patients about their condition, treatment options, and the importance of adherence to therapy.

3. How To Use This Book

A. Overview Of The Book's Structure

Chapter Breakdown:

Introduction and Background: Initial chapters provide an overview of H. pylori, its impact on health, and the book's objectives.

Diagnosis: Detailed information on diagnostic methods and how to interpret results.

Treatment: Comprehensive coverage of treatment strategies, including medications and management practices.

Lifestyle and Management: Practical advice for patients on managing symptoms and making lifestyle changes.

Special Sections:

Case Studies: Real-life case studies and examples to illustrate different aspects of diagnosis and treatment.

FAQs and Troubleshooting: Sections addressing common questions and issues encountered in managing H. pylori infections.

B. Tips For Navigating The Content

Use the Table of Contents:

Find Relevant Information: Use the table of contents to locate specific topics of interest, whether you are seeking information on diagnosis, treatment, or management strategies.

Refer to Index:

Quick Access: Utilize the index to quickly find information on particular terms or topics related to H. pylori.

Consult Appendices:

Additional Resources: Review appendices for supplementary information, including diagnostic criteria, treatment guidelines, and additional resources for further reading.

Apply Practical Advice:

Real-World Application: Apply the practical advice provided to both patient and healthcare provider scenarios for effective management of H. pylori infections.

CHAPTER 1: UNDERSTANDING H. PYLORI

What Is H. Pylori?

Bacterial Characteristics And Lifecycle

Common Symptoms And Associated Conditions (E.G., Peptic Ulcers, Gastritis)

Transmission And Risk Factors

How H. Pylori Spreads

Risk Factors For Infection

Diagnosis

Symptoms Prompting Testing

Diagnostic Methods (Breath Test, Stool Test, Blood Test, Endoscopy With Biopsy)

Helicobacter pylori (H. pylori) is a significant pathogen in gastrointestinal health, known for its role in various stomach-related conditions. This section will explore what H. pylori is, how it spreads and what increases the risk of infection, and the methods used to diagnose it.

1. What Is H. Pylori?

A. Bacterial Characteristics And Lifecycle

Bacterial Characteristics:

Shape and Structure: H. pylori is a spiral-shaped, gram-negative bacterium. Its unique spiral form helps it navigate through the thick mucus lining of the stomach.

Motility: It has flagella that allow it to move through the viscous stomach environment, which aids in its survival and colonization.

Survival Mechanisms: H. pylori produces urease, an enzyme that breaks down urea into ammonia and carbon dioxide. This neutralizes stomach acid in its immediate environment, creating a more hospitable niche for the bacterium.

Lifecycle:

Colonization: After entering the stomach, H. pylori adheres to the gastric epithelium, where it evades the immune response and survives in the acidic environment.

Inflammation: The presence of H. pylori triggers chronic inflammation of the stomach lining, known as chronic gastritis. This inflammation can disrupt normal gastric function and lead to various symptoms and complications.

Long-Term Effects: If left untreated, H. pylori infection can persist for years or even decades, potentially leading to more severe conditions such as peptic ulcers or gastric cancer.

B. Common Symptoms And Associated Conditions

Common Symptoms:

Abdominal Pain: Persistent or recurring pain in the upper abdomen is common. It may be described as burning or gnawing.

Nausea and Vomiting: Infected individuals may experience nausea, which can sometimes lead to vomiting.

Bloating and Burping: Symptoms like bloating, excessive burping, or a feeling of fullness can occur.

Loss of Appetite: Decreased appetite and unintentional weight loss may also be present.

Associated Conditions:

Peptic Ulcers: H. pylori is a major cause of peptic ulcers, which are sores that develop on the lining of the stomach, small intestine, or esophagus. Symptoms include pain, bloating, and indigestion.

Chronic Gastritis: Chronic inflammation of the stomach lining due to H. pylori can lead to symptoms such as abdominal pain and nausea. Over time, it can affect digestion and stomach function.

Gastric Cancer: Long-term infection with H. pylori increases the risk of developing gastric cancer, particularly in individuals with chronic gastritis or a family history of the disease.

2. Transmission And Risk Factors

A. How H. Pylori Spreads

Transmission Routes:

Oral-Fecal Transmission: H. pylori is commonly spread through the oral-fecal route. This can occur via contaminated food or water, especially in areas with poor sanitation.

Oral-Oral Transmission: The bacterium may also spread through direct contact with saliva, such as through kissing or sharing utensils.

Environmental Factors:

Sanitation: Poor hygiene and inadequate sanitation contribute to the spread of H. pylori. Infected individuals can transmit the bacteria to others through contaminated food or water.

Living Conditions: Crowded living conditions and close contact with infected individuals increase the likelihood of transmission.

B. Risk Factors For Infection

Demographic Factors:

Age: H. pylori infection is more common in childhood, especially in developing countries where sanitation may be lacking. However, it can occur at any age.

Geographic Region: The prevalence of H. pylori varies by region, with higher rates often seen in developing countries compared to developed nations.

Lifestyle and Health Factors:

Socioeconomic Status: Individuals from lower socioeconomic backgrounds are at higher risk due to factors such as poor sanitation and crowded living conditions.

Family History: A family history of H. pylori infection or related gastrointestinal conditions may increase an individual's risk.

Immune System Status: People with compromised immune systems or other underlying health conditions may be more susceptible to H. pylori infection and its complications.

3. Diagnosis

A. Symptoms Prompting Testing

When to Seek Testing:

Persistent Symptoms: Individuals experiencing chronic symptoms such as abdominal pain, nausea, bloating, and loss of appetite should consider testing for H. pylori.

Severe Conditions: Those with suspected peptic ulcers, chronic gastritis, or unexplained weight loss should seek diagnosis and management.

Routine Screening:

High-Risk Individuals: Regular screening may be recommended for individuals with a family history of gastric cancer or other risk factors for H. pylori-related diseases.

B. Diagnostic Methods

Breath Test:

Procedure: The urea breath test involves drinking a liquid containing a substance that

H. pylori breaks down. The resulting carbon dioxide is measured in the breath to indicate the presence of the bacterium.

Advantages: Non-invasive and highly accurate for detecting active infection.

Stool Test:

Procedure: A stool sample is analyzed for the presence of H. pylori antigens, which indicates an active infection.

Advantages: Convenient and non-invasive, suitable for detecting ongoing infection.

Blood Test:

Procedure: A blood sample is tested for antibodies against H. pylori. This test can indicate past or current infection but is less effective for diagnosing active infections.

Advantages: Useful for initial screening but less specific than other methods.

Endoscopy with Biopsy:

Procedure: An endoscopic examination involves inserting a thin, flexible tube with a camera into the stomach to visualize the lining and obtain biopsy samples for testing.

Advantages: Provides direct visualization and allows for biopsy, which can confirm the presence of H. pylori and assess damage to the stomach lining.

CHAPTER 2: CONVENTIONAL TREATMENT APPROACHES

Antibiotic Therapy

Commonly Used Antibiotics (E.G., Amoxicillin, Clarithromycin, Metronidazole)

Regimens And Duration

Side Effects And Considerations

Proton Pump Inhibitors (Ppis)

Role In Treatment

Examples (E.G., Omeprazole, Lansoprazole)

Dosage And Potential Side Effects

Bismuth Subsalicylate

Use In Combination Therapy

Benefits And Possible Side Effects

Treatment Protocols

Standard Triple Therapy

Quadruple Therapy

Effective treatment of Helicobacter pylori (H. pylori) infections typically involves a combination of antibiotics and medications to reduce stomach acid. This section covers the key components of conventional treatment approaches, including commonly used antibiotics, proton pump inhibitors (PPIs), bismuth subsalicylate, and standard treatment protocols.

1. Antibiotic Therapy

A. Commonly Used Antibiotics

Amoxicillin: Function: Amoxicillin is a broad-spectrum penicillin antibiotic that targets and kills H. pylori bacteria.

Dosage: Typically administered 1 gram twice daily.

Administration: Often used in combination with other antibiotics and medications to enhance efficacy.

Clarithromycin:

Function: Clarithromycin is a macrolide antibiotic that inhibits bacterial protein synthesis, which helps eradicate H. pylori.

Dosage: Commonly prescribed 500 mg twice daily.

Administration: Often paired with amoxicillin and a PPI for a comprehensive treatment regimen.

Metronidazole:

Function: Metronidazole is an antibiotic with anaerobic activity, effective against H. pylori in conjunction with other drugs.

Dosage: Typically 500 mg twice or three times daily.

Administration: Used in combination therapies, especially if there is resistance to other antibiotics.

B. Regimens And Duration

Regimens:

Standard Triple Therapy: Involves a combination of two antibiotics (commonly amoxicillin and clarithromycin) and a proton pump inhibitor (PPI) for 10-14 days.

Quadruple Therapy: Combines two antibiotics (e.g., metronidazole and tetracycline), a PPI, and bismuth subsalicylate, usually for 10-14 days. This approach is often used when resistance to standard therapy is suspected or confirmed.

Duration:

Typical Duration: Treatment courses generally last between 10 to 14 days. Adherence to the full course is crucial to effectively eradicate the infection and reduce the risk of resistance.

C. Side Effects And Considerations

Common Side Effects:

Antibiotics: May include gastrointestinal symptoms such as nausea, vomiting, diarrhea, and allergic reactions.

Metronidazole: May cause a metallic taste, nausea, and potential interactions with alcohol (disulfiram-like reaction).

Considerations:

Allergies: Patients with penicillin allergies should avoid amoxicillin and consider alternative antibiotics.

Drug Interactions: Be aware of potential interactions with other medications and adjust treatment accordingly.

2. Proton Pump Inhibitors (Ppis)

A. Role In Treatment

Function: PPIs reduce stomach acid production, which helps in healing the stomach lining and enhances the effectiveness of antibiotics by creating a less acidic environment for the medications to work.

Impact: They help alleviate symptoms such as heartburn and gastric pain associated with H. pylori infection.

B. Examples

Omeprazole:

Dosage: Typically 20 mg to 40 mg once daily.

Administration: Commonly used in combination with antibiotics and sometimes bismuth subsalicylate.

Lansoprazole:

Dosage: Usually 15 mg to 30 mg once daily.

Administration: Often included in treatment regimens for its effectiveness in reducing acid production.

C. Dosage And Potential Side Effects

Dosage:

General Recommendation: PPIs are usually administered once or twice daily, depending on the specific drug and treatment regimen.

Potential Side Effects:

Common Effects: May include headache, nausea, diarrhea, and abdominal pain.

Long-Term Use: Prolonged use of PPIs can lead to side effects such as increased risk of bone fractures, kidney disease, and gastrointestinal infections.

3. Bismuth Subsalicylate

A. Use In Combination Therapy

Function: Bismuth subsalicylate is used in combination therapy to help with eradication of H. pylori and to provide additional anti-inflammatory effects.

Benefit: It has antimicrobial properties that complement the effects of antibiotics and PPIs in H. pylori treatment regimens.

B. Benefits And Possible Side Effects

Benefits:

Additional Support: Helps in reducing symptoms such as nausea and upset stomach.

Enhanced Eradication: Can improve the effectiveness of the overall treatment regimen.

Possible Side Effects:

Common Effects: Black stool and tongue, mild gastrointestinal discomfort.

Rare Effects: Allergic reactions, especially in individuals with salicylate sensitivity.

4. Treatment Protocols

A. Standard Triple Therapy

Components: Typically includes two antibiotics (e.g., amoxicillin and clarithromycin) and a PPI.

Duration: Usually administered for 10-14 days.

Effectiveness: Effective in many cases but may be less effective in areas with high rates of antibiotic resistance.

b. Quadruple Therapy

Components: Includes two antibiotics (e.g., metronidazole and tetracycline), a PPI, and bismuth subsalicylate.

Duration: Generally 10-14 days.

Effectiveness: Often used when there is resistance to triple therapy or in cases of treatment failure.

C. Factors Influencing Treatment Choice

Antibiotic Resistance:

Testing: Resistance testing may be performed to tailor the treatment to the specific strain of H. pylori.

Adaptation: Treatment may need to be adjusted based on resistance patterns in the local population.

Patient History:

Prior Treatments: Previous treatments and their outcomes can influence the choice of therapy.

Comorbid Conditions: Other health conditions and medications may affect treatment decisions.

CHAPTER 3: MANAGING TREATMENT-RESISTANT H. PYLORI

Understanding Antibiotic Resistance

How Resistance Develops

Impact On Treatment Efficacy

Alternative Treatment Strategies

Different Antibiotic Combinations

Role Of Salvage Therapy

Monitoring And Follow-Up

Importance Of Follow-Up Testing

Managing Persistent Or Recurrent Infection

When H. pylori infections prove resistant to initial treatment regimens, it's crucial to understand the underlying issues and explore alternative strategies. This section addresses the development of antibiotic resistance, alternative treatment strategies, and the importance of monitoring and follow-up.

1. Understanding Antibiotic Resistance

A. How Resistance Develops

Mechanisms of Resistance:

Genetic Mutations: H. pylori can develop genetic mutations that alter its susceptibility to antibiotics. These mutations may affect drug-targeted sites, reducing drug effectiveness.

Enzymatic Breakdown: The bacteria can produce enzymes, such as beta-lactamases, that break down antibiotics like amoxicillin, rendering them ineffective.

Efflux Pumps: Some strains use efflux pumps to expel antibiotics from the bacterial cell before they can exert their effects.

Contributing Factors:

Inappropriate Use: Overuse or incorrect use of antibiotics can lead to resistance. This includes incomplete courses of antibiotics and unnecessary prescriptions.

Previous Treatments: Prior exposure to antibiotics can select for resistant strains if the full course of treatment was not completed or if the antibiotics were not appropriately targeted.

B. Impact On Treatment Efficacy

Reduced Effectiveness:

Failure of Standard Regimens: Antibiotic resistance can lead to the failure of standard triple or quadruple therapy, necessitating alternative approaches.

Persistent Symptoms: Patients may continue to experience symptoms such as abdominal pain, nausea, and dyspepsia if the infection is not fully eradicated.

Complications:

Increased Risk of Complications: Persistent H. pylori infection can exacerbate conditions like peptic ulcers and gastritis, potentially leading to more severe gastrointestinal issues.

Long-Term Health Effects: Continued infection may have long-term effects on gastrointestinal health and increase the risk of gastric cancer.

2. Alternative Treatment Strategies

A. Different Antibiotic Combinations

Revised Antibiotic Regimens:

Alternative Antibiotics: If resistance to first-line antibiotics is suspected, alternative antibiotics such as levofloxacin, moxifloxacin, or rifabutin may be used. The choice depends on local resistance patterns and prior treatments.

Adjusting Dosage: Dosages may be adjusted based on the specific antibiotics used and patient tolerance.

Tailored Therapy:

Sensitivity Testing: Antibiotic sensitivity testing can identify which antibiotics are effective against the specific H. pylori strain in a patient, allowing for more targeted treatment.

Customized Regimens: Based on sensitivity results, a customized regimen combining effective antibiotics with a PPI can be designed.

b. Role of Salvage Therapy

Definition and Purpose:

Salvage Therapy: This is a treatment approach used after failure of initial therapy. It often includes a combination of antibiotics not used in the first-line treatment, along with a PPI and sometimes bismuth subsalicylate.

Objective: The goal is to eradicate H. pylori using a regimen that has a different mechanism of action or uses antibiotics to which the bacteria have not developed resistance.

Examples of Salvage Therapy:

Levofloxacin-Based Regimen: Includes levofloxacin, amoxicillin, and a PPI, used when resistance to clarithromycin is present.

Bismuth Quadruple Therapy: Combines bismuth subsalicylate, metronidazole, tetracycline, and a PPI, which is effective against many resistant strains.

3. Monitoring And Follow-Up

A. Importance Of Follow-Up Testing
Confirming Eradication:

Testing Methods: After completing a treatment regimen, tests such as the urea breath test, stool antigen test, or endoscopy with biopsy are used to confirm that H. pylori has been eradicated.

Timing of Tests: Follow-up testing is usually performed at least 4 weeks after the completion of therapy to avoid false negatives due to residual antibiotics.

Avoiding Reinfection:

Lifestyle and Hygiene: Patients should be advised on preventive measures, such as good hygiene and avoiding contaminated food and water, to reduce the risk of reinfection.

B. Managing Persistent Or Recurrent Infection

Reassessment and Adjustment:

Reviewing Treatment History: If symptoms persist or recur, a thorough review of previous treatments, including antibiotic regimens and adherence, is necessary.

Revised Testing: Additional testing may be required to identify any new resistance patterns or underlying conditions contributing to the infection.

Alternative Approaches:

Consultation with Specialists: In cases of persistent infection, consultation with a gastroenterologist or an infectious disease specialist may be necessary for advanced management and treatment strategies.

Long-Term Monitoring: Ongoing monitoring and adjustments to treatment plans can help manage chronic or recurrent cases effectively.

CHAPTER 4: INTEGRATIVE AND COMPLEMENTARY THERAPIES

Diet And Lifestyle Adjustments

Foods To Avoid And Foods To Include

Impact Of Diet On Treatment And Healing

Probiotics And Prebiotics

Role In Gut Health And H. Pylori Treatment

Recommended Strains And Dosages

Herbal And Natural Remedies

Efficacy And Safety Of Various Herbs And Supplements

Research Findings And Clinical Evidence
Integrative and complementary therapies can play a supportive role in managing H. pylori infections and enhancing overall gastrointestinal health. This section explores dietary and lifestyle adjustments,

the use of probiotics and prebiotics, and the efficacy of herbal and natural remedies.

1. Diet And Lifestyle Adjustments

A. Foods To Avoid And Foods To Include

Foods to Avoid:

Spicy Foods: Can exacerbate gastritis and ulcer symptoms. Examples include chili peppers, hot sauces, and heavily spiced dishes.

Acidic Foods and Beverages: Citrus fruits, tomatoes, and carbonated drinks can irritate the stomach lining.

High-Fat Foods: Fried foods and those high in saturated fats can increase gastric acid production and aggravate symptoms.

Alcohol and Caffeine: Both can irritate the gastrointestinal tract and may interfere with treatment.

Foods to Include:

Non-Irritating, Low-Acidity Foods: Bananas, oatmeal, and cooked vegetables are gentle on the stomach.

Foods Rich in Fiber: Whole grains, fruits, and vegetables can support overall digestive health and may aid in reducing symptoms.

Lean Proteins: Chicken, fish, and tofu are good sources of protein without adding excessive fat.

Antioxidant-Rich Foods: Berries, leafy greens, and nuts can help reduce inflammation and support healing.

B. Impact Of Diet On Treatment And Healing

Symptom Relief:

Soothing Foods: Consuming bland, soothing foods can reduce discomfort and aid in healing the gastric mucosa.

Reduced Acid Production: A diet low in acidic and irritating foods can help minimize gastric acid production, which may alleviate symptoms.

Support for Treatment:

Nutrient Absorption: Proper nutrition supports overall health and ensures that the body can effectively utilize medications and treatments.

Enhanced Healing: Nutrients from a balanced diet can aid in the repair of the stomach lining and support immune function.

2. Probiotics And Prebiotics

A. Role In Gut Health And H. Pylori Treatment

Probiotics:

Gut Flora Balance: Probiotics can help restore the balance of gut bacteria, which may be disrupted by H. pylori and its treatment. This can potentially improve symptoms and support healing.

Reduction of Side Effects: They may reduce gastrointestinal side effects associated with antibiotic therapy, such as diarrhea and dysbiosis.

Prebiotics:

Support for Probiotics: Prebiotics are non-digestible fibers that promote the growth of beneficial bacteria in the gut. They can enhance the effectiveness of probiotics and contribute to a healthy gut microbiome.

Symptom Management: By fostering a healthy gut environment, prebiotics may help improve symptoms and support overall digestive health.

B. Recommended Strains And Dosages

Probiotic Strains:

Lactobacillus species (e.g., Lactobacillus acidophilus): Known for their ability to survive in the gastrointestinal tract and support gut health.

Bifidobacterium species (e.g., Bifidobacterium bifidum): Help in maintaining a balanced gut microbiome and may alleviate gastrointestinal symptoms.

Saccharomyces boulardii: A yeast probiotic that may help reduce antibiotic-associated diarrhea and support gut health.

Dosages:

General Recommendations: A typical dosage ranges from 1 to 10 billion CFUs (colony-forming units) per day, but this can vary based on the specific strain and product.

Consultation with a Healthcare Provider: It's essential to consult with a healthcare provider for personalized recommendations and to address any specific health concerns.

3. Herbal And Natural Remedies

A. Efficacy And Safety Of Various Herbs And Supplements

Herbal Remedies:

Ginger: Known for its anti-inflammatory and digestive properties. It may help soothe gastrointestinal discomfort and nausea.

Garlic: Has antimicrobial properties and may support gut health by potentially reducing H. pylori activity.

Green Tea: Contains antioxidants that may help reduce inflammation and support digestive health.

Supplements:

Licorice Root: Can have anti-inflammatory and healing effects on the gastrointestinal mucosa but should be used cautiously due to potential side effects.

Slippery Elm: Contains mucilage that can coat and soothe the stomach lining, potentially providing symptom relief.

B. Research Findings And Clinical Evidence

Studies on Herbal Remedies:

Efficacy: Some studies suggest that certain herbs, like garlic and ginger, may have beneficial effects on gastrointestinal health and may support traditional treatment for H. pylori.

Evidence: Clinical evidence is mixed, and while some herbal remedies show promise, they should be used as complementary rather than primary treatments.

Safety Considerations:

Side Effects: Herbal supplements can interact with medications and may have side effects. It's crucial to discuss their use with a healthcare provider.

Quality Control: Ensure that herbal products are sourced from reputable manufacturers to avoid contaminants and ensure efficacy.

CHAPTER 5: LIFESTYLE AND PREVENTION

Preventing H. Pylori Infection

Hygiene Practices And Preventive Measures

Importance Of Clean Water And Food

Managing Symptoms And Complications

Strategies For Alleviating Symptoms Like Nausea, Pain, And Bloating

Addressing Complications Like Ulcers Or Gastritis

Long-Term Health Considerations

Monitoring For Long-Term Effects Of H. Pylori Infection

Managing Potential Chronic Conditions

Managing and preventing H. pylori infection involves understanding how to minimize the risk of infection, addressing symptoms effectively, and being aware of long-term health considerations. This section provides practical strategies for preventing infection, managing symptoms and complications, and considering long-term health impacts.

1. Preventing H. Pylori Infection

A. Hygiene Practices And Preventive Measures

Hand Hygiene:

Regular Hand Washing: Wash hands thoroughly with soap and water, especially before eating or preparing food and after using the restroom.

Hand Sanitizers: Use alcohol-based hand sanitizers when soap and water are not available, though washing with soap and water is preferable.

Food Safety:

Proper Cooking: Ensure all meats are cooked thoroughly to kill any potential bacteria. This is particularly important for poultry and ground meats.

Avoid Cross-Contamination: Use separate cutting boards and utensils for raw meat and ready-to-eat foods. Clean surfaces and utensils with hot, soapy water after use.

Food Storage: Store food at the correct temperatures to prevent bacterial growth. Refrigerate perishable items promptly and properly.

Safe Water Consumption:

Drink Clean Water: Use filtered or bottled water if the source of tap water is questionable. Ensure water is from a safe and reliable source.

Avoid Contaminated Water: Be cautious with water from unreliable sources, especially when traveling in areas with poor sanitation.

B. Importance Of Clean Water And Food

Prevention of Infection:

Clean Water: Contaminated water can be a source of H. pylori and other pathogens. Ensuring access to clean, treated water helps reduce the risk of infection.

Food Safety: Proper food handling and preparation minimize the risk of bacterial contamination and transmission.

Health Promotion:

Overall Health: Good hygiene and food safety practices contribute to general health and well-being, reducing the likelihood of gastrointestinal infections.

2. Managing Symptoms And Complications

A. Strategies For Alleviating Symptoms

Nausea and Pain:

Dietary Adjustments: Eat small, frequent meals and avoid spicy, fatty, or acidic foods that can exacerbate nausea and pain. Opt for bland, soothing foods like rice, applesauce, and toast.

Hydration: Drink plenty of fluids to stay hydrated, especially if experiencing vomiting or diarrhea.

Bloating:

Avoid Gas-Producing Foods: Limit intake of foods that can cause gas and bloating, such as beans, carbonated beverages, and cruciferous vegetables.

Eating Habits: Eat slowly and chew food thoroughly to reduce swallowed air and improve digestion.

B. Addressing Complications

Ulcers:

Medication: Use prescribed medications, such as proton pump inhibitors (PPIs) or H2-receptor antagonists, to reduce stomach acid and promote ulcer healing.

Avoid Irritants: Refrain from using nonsteroidal anti-inflammatory drugs (NSAIDs) and other irritants that can worsen ulcers.

Gastritis:

Treatment: Follow prescribed treatments to manage inflammation of the stomach lining, including medications and dietary changes.

Avoid Triggers: Identify and avoid foods and substances that trigger gastritis symptoms.

3. Long-Term Health Considerations

A. Monitoring For Long-Term Effects

Regular Check-Ups:

Gastroenterological Assessments: Regular visits to a gastroenterologist can help monitor for any long-term effects of H. pylori infection, such as chronic gastritis or ulcers.

Screening: Periodic testing may be necessary to ensure that H. pylori has been eradicated and to check for any recurring infection.

Symptom Management:

Ongoing Symptoms: Manage any persistent symptoms with appropriate medical guidance and lifestyle modifications to ensure quality of life.

B. Managing Potential Chronic Conditions

Chronic Gastric Conditions:

Long-Term Treatment: Individuals who have developed chronic conditions due to H. pylori infection may need long-term treatment and monitoring to manage these conditions effectively.

Diet and Lifestyle: Continue to adhere to dietary and lifestyle adjustments to support overall gastric health and prevent complications.

General Health Maintenance:

Healthy Habits: Maintain a balanced diet, engage in regular physical activity, and practice good hygiene to support overall health and prevent other potential health issues.

CHAPTER 6: NAVIGATING THE HEALTHCARE SYSTEM

Choosing A Healthcare Provider

Roles Of Gastroenterologists And Primary Care Physicians

How To Find A Specialist

Insurance And Financial Aspects

Coverage For Diagnostic Tests And Treatments

Financial Assistance And Support Resources

Patient Advocacy And Rights

Understanding Patient Rights

How To Advocate For Your Health

Effectively navigating the healthcare system is crucial for managing H. pylori infections and ensuring you receive the appropriate diagnosis, treatment, and support. This section outlines how to choose the right healthcare provider, understand insurance and financial aspects, and advocate for your health.

1. Choosing A Healthcare Provider

A. Roles Of Gastroenterologists And Primary Care Physicians

Primary Care Physicians (PCPs):

Initial Evaluation: PCPs are often the first point of contact for patients with gastrointestinal symptoms. They can provide initial assessments, manage routine care, and refer patients to specialists if necessary.

Long-Term Management: They can coordinate overall health care and manage other aspects of health that may be affected by or related to H. pylori infection.

Gastroenterologists:

Specialized Care: Gastroenterologists specialize in diagnosing and treating gastrointestinal disorders, including H. pylori infections. They have expertise in advanced diagnostic procedures and treatment options.

Advanced Diagnostics: They perform specialized tests, such as endoscopy with biopsy, and can offer targeted therapies for complex or resistant H. pylori infections.

B. How To Find A Specialist

Referrals:

Ask Your PCP: Your primary care physician can provide referrals to experienced gastroenterologists based on your specific needs and location.

Consult Insurance Networks: Check with your health insurance provider for a list of in-network gastroenterologists to reduce out-of-pocket costs.

Online Resources:

Medical Websites: Use websites like the American College of Gastroenterology (ACG) or the American Gastroenterological Association (AGA) to find certified specialists.

Patient Reviews: Look for reviews and ratings on healthcare review sites to get an idea of other patients' experiences with a particular specialist.

Professional Associations:

Gastroenterology Associations: Membership in professional associations can indicate a specialist's commitment to ongoing education and adherence to best practices.

2. Insurance And Financial Aspects

A. Coverage For Diagnostic Tests And Treatments

Understanding Your Plan:

Review Benefits: Examine your health insurance plan to understand coverage details for diagnostic tests (e.g., breath tests, endoscopy) and treatments (e.g., antibiotics, proton pump inhibitors).

In-Network vs. Out-of-Network: Confirm whether the diagnostic tests and treatments are covered if performed by in-network versus out-of-network providers.

Pre-Authorization and Referrals:

Pre-Authorization: Some insurance plans require pre-authorization for certain procedures or treatments. Ensure that your healthcare provider obtains any necessary approvals before proceeding.

Referrals: If required by your insurance plan, obtain referrals from your primary care physician before seeing a specialist.

B. Financial Assistance And Support Resources

Patient Assistance Programs:

Pharmaceutical Companies: Many drug manufacturers offer patient assistance programs that provide financial aid or discounts for prescription medications.

Nonprofits: Organizations like the American Gastroenterological Association (AGA) may offer resources or support for managing healthcare costs.

Health Savings Accounts (HSAs) and Flexible Spending Accounts (FSAs):

Tax Benefits: Use HSAs or FSAs to pay for eligible medical expenses with pre-tax dollars, potentially reducing out-of-pocket costs.

Payment Plans:

Negotiation: Discuss payment plan options with healthcare providers if you face difficulty covering treatment costs. Some providers offer flexible payment arrangements.

3. Patient Advocacy and Rights

a. Understanding Patient Rights

Access to Care:

Right to Information: Patients have the right to receive clear and accurate information about their diagnosis, treatment options, and prognosis.

Informed Consent: Ensure you understand the risks and benefits of treatments and procedures and provide informed consent before any interventions.

Confidentiality:

Privacy: Your medical information should be kept confidential according to privacy laws such as HIPAA (Health Insurance Portability and Accountability Act).

Right to Quality Care:

Non-Discrimination: You have the right to receive care without discrimination based on race, gender, socioeconomic status, or other factors.

b. How to Advocate for Your Health

Communication:

Be Proactive: Clearly communicate your symptoms, concerns, and questions to your healthcare providers. Don't hesitate to seek clarification on anything you don't understand.

Follow-Up: Regularly follow up on treatment plans, appointments, and test results to stay informed about your health status.

Seek a Second Opinion:

Alternative Perspectives: If you're uncertain about a diagnosis or treatment plan, consider seeking a second opinion from another specialist to confirm the recommended approach.

Patient Advocacy Groups:

Support and Resources: Engage with patient advocacy organizations that offer support, educational resources, and assistance in navigating the healthcare system.

Document Your Health Care:

Keep Records: Maintain thorough records of your medical history, treatments, and communications with healthcare providers. This documentation can be valuable for managing your care and resolving any issues.

CHAPTER 7: FUTURE DIRECTIONS IN H. PYLORI RESEARCH

Ongoing Research And Clinical Trials

Areas Of Current Research

How To Participate In Trials

Innovations In Treatment

New Therapies And Drug Developments

Advances In Diagnostic Technologies

The Future Of H. Pylori Management

Predictions And Emerging Trends

Potential For Eradication And Improved Treatment Approaches

The ongoing advancements in H. pylori research aim to enhance our understanding of the infection, develop more effective treatments, and ultimately improve patient outcomes. This section explores current research areas, emerging innovations in treatment, and future trends in H. pylori management.

1. Ongoing Research And Clinical Trials

A. Areas Of Current Research

Mechanisms of Pathogenesis:

Understanding Virulence Factors: Researchers are studying how H. pylori interacts with the host's immune system and contributes to disease progression. Identifying specific virulence factors could lead to targeted therapies.

Microbiome Interactions: Investigating how H. pylori affects and is affected by the gut microbiome, and how these interactions impact disease and treatment responses.

Antibiotic Resistance:

Resistance Mechanisms: Research is focusing on the genetic and biochemical mechanisms behind antibiotic resistance in H. pylori, which could help in developing strategies to overcome this challenge.

New Antimicrobial Agents: Exploring novel antibiotics or alternative agents that are effective against resistant strains of H. pylori.

Long-Term Effects:

Chronic Conditions: Studying the long-term health impacts of H. pylori infection, including its role in chronic diseases like gastric cancer or peptic ulcers.

Post-Treatment Outcomes: Evaluating the effectiveness of current treatments in the long term and identifying factors that contribute to recurrence.

B. How To Participate In Trials

Finding Clinical Trials:

ClinicalTrials.gov: Use this database to search for ongoing H. pylori research trials. It provides information on trial locations, eligibility criteria, and contact details.

Research Institutions: Contact local research hospitals or universities that conduct clinical trials related to gastroenterology or infectious diseases.

Eligibility and Enrollment:

Screening Process: Trials often have specific inclusion and exclusion criteria. Understand these requirements and discuss them with your healthcare provider.

Informed Consent: Ensure you fully understand the potential risks and benefits before participating. Read and sign an informed consent document that outlines the study's purpose and procedures.

Patient Advocacy Groups:

Support Networks: Engage with advocacy organizations that provide information on clinical trials and support participants throughout the research process.

2. Innovations In Treatment

A. New Therapies And Drug Developments

Novel Antibiotics:

Emerging Drugs: Researchers are developing new antibiotics specifically targeting H. pylori with improved efficacy and reduced resistance. Examples include new classes of drugs or modifications of existing antibiotics.

Bacteriophage Therapy:

Phage Therapy: This innovative approach involves using bacteriophages (viruses that infect bacteria) to target and kill H. pylori. Early research shows promise in overcoming antibiotic resistance.

Vaccines:

Preventive Vaccines: Development of vaccines to prevent H. pylori infection is underway. These vaccines could potentially reduce the incidence of infection and its associated complications.

b. Advances in Diagnostic Technologies
Molecular Diagnostics:

Genetic Testing: Advances in molecular diagnostics include testing for specific genetic markers of H. pylori and its resistance patterns, allowing for more personalized treatment approaches.

Non-Invasive Testing:

Breath and Stool Tests: Improved accuracy and convenience of non-invasive diagnostic tests, such as urea breath tests and stool antigen tests, to detect H. pylori infection more reliably.

Endoscopic Innovations:

Enhanced Imaging: New technologies in endoscopy, such as high-resolution imaging and narrow-band imaging, are being developed to better visualize and biopsy infected areas in the gastrointestinal tract.

3. The Future Of H. Pylori Management

A. Predictions And Emerging Trends

Personalized Medicine:

Tailored Treatments: Future management of H. pylori infection may involve personalized treatment plans based on individual genetic profiles, resistance patterns, and disease progression.

Integrated Care Models:

Holistic Approaches: Incorporating multidisciplinary approaches that combine pharmacological treatments, lifestyle modifications, and integrative therapies for comprehensive management of H. pylori.

Global Health Initiatives:

Public Health Campaigns: Increased focus on global health strategies to manage and prevent H. pylori infections in regions where it is endemic, with efforts to improve sanitation and education.

B. Potential For Eradication And Improved Treatment Approaches

Eradication Efforts:

Global Eradication Goals: Research aims to develop strategies for the potential eradication of H. pylori, similar to successful eradication programs for other infectious diseases.

Enhanced Treatment Protocols:

New Regimens: Development of more effective treatment regimens with shorter durations and fewer side effects to increase patient adherence and success rates.

Long-Term Management:

Preventive Strategies: Emphasis on preventive measures and monitoring to reduce recurrence rates and manage chronic conditions related to H. pylori.

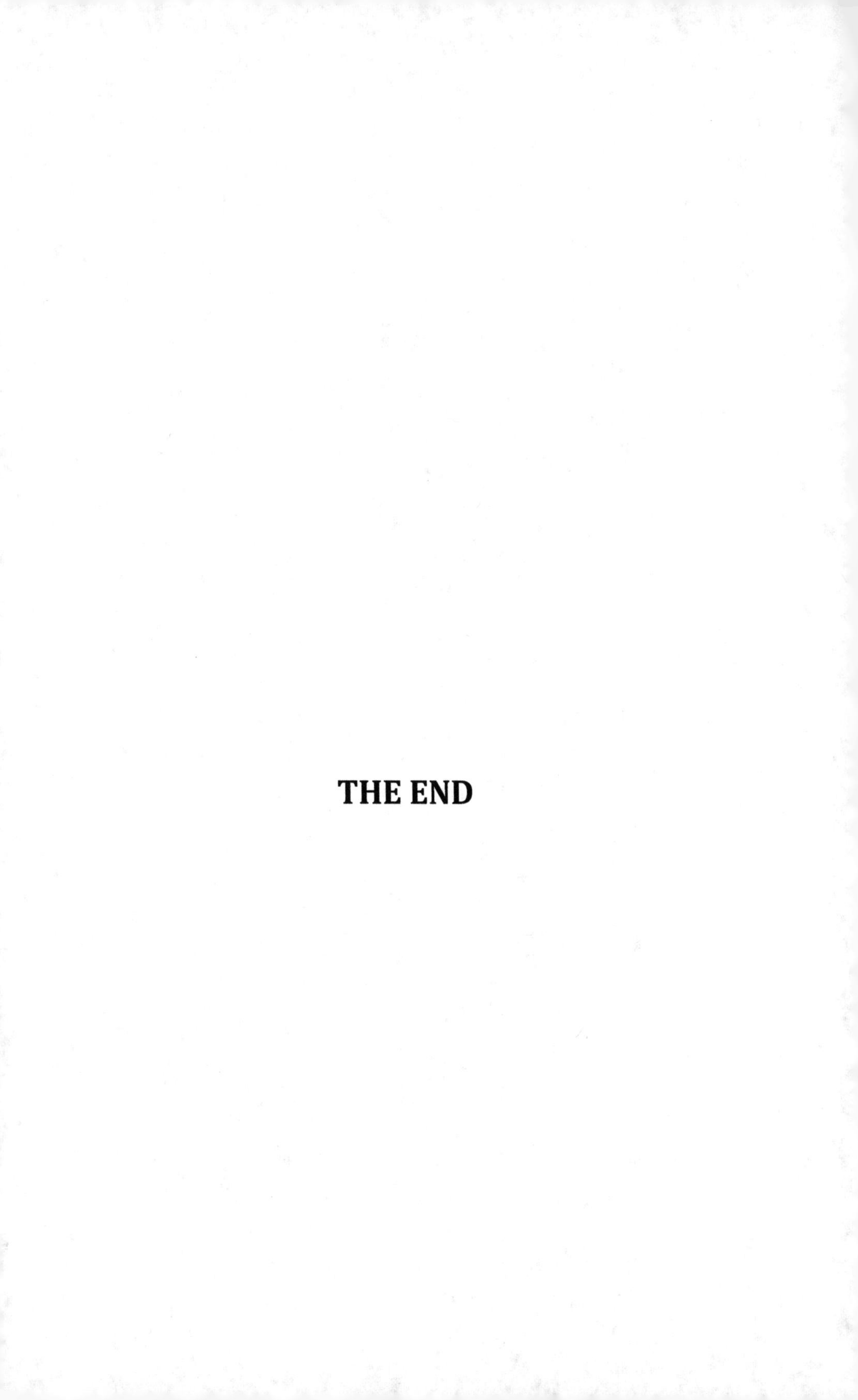

THE END